Trigger Point Therapy
Routine for TMJ

— Massage Techniques to Unlock Your TMJ —

Annie Coomes LMT, CST
Illustrated by Christine Kenney MScBMC

Balboa Press books may be ordered through booksellers or by contacting:

Balboa Press
A Division of Hay House
1663 Liberty Drive
Bloomington, IN 47403
www.balboapress.com
1 (877) 407-4847

Because of the dynamic nature of the Internet, any web addresses or links contained in this book may have changed since publication and may no longer be valid. The views expressed in this work are solely those of the author and do not necessarily reflect the views of the publisher, and the publisher hereby disclaims any responsibility for them.

Any people depicted in stock imagery provided by Thinkstock are models, and such images are being used for illustrative purposes only.
Certain stock imagery © Thinkstock.

ISBN: 978-1-5043-7410-1 (sc)
ISBN: 978-1-5043-7409-5 (e)

Print information available on the last page.

Balboa Press rev. date: 03/30/2017

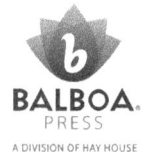

BALBOA
PRESS
A DIVISION OF HAY HOUSE

CONTENTS

For my clients through the years who have trusted the inherent wisdom in the body, your trust has deeply touched my soul and reinforced my passion for this work, and you have been my greatest teachers.

PREFACE

This book has come into being through the requests of my clients through the years. They have seen the benefits of this routine. They have brought in their children when the dentist was talking about braces or removing teeth to make room. This routine, along with craniosacral therapy, opened up and realigned the muscles and bones so some children did not have to go through the event of wearing braces.

This routine has many applications. Who benefits?

- Those seeking relief after dental and orthodontic visits
- Children and adults that grind or clench their teeth
- Children and teens wearing braces, the routine can help between dental visits to relieve tension
- Those who have ringing in the ears and sinus problems
- Sleep apnea patients and denture wearers
- Headaches and migraines
- Facial nerve pain and ticks

At one time or another, all my clients have experienced this routine.

There will always be a need for temporomandibular joint (TMJ) work. The constant use of the jaw when talking and chewing alone will reinforce the need for this routine. I think the most important opportunity is to work with our children and teach them this routine is of the utmost importance. We can start to educate them on taking care of their bodies and see how much better they can feel with preventative therapy.

We can start by massaging our babies and helping to reduce the tension and stress from birth. Massage strengthens bonding, sensory development in the nervous system and communication with baby. How wonderful to have massage from such an early age. As our children grow, they will learn the power of touch and the healing capabilities it has for our mental emotional and physical well-being. And hopefully they will pass on this healing touch to their children.

INTRODUCTION

Welcome to the world of massage therapy and bodywork, an alternative treatment that brings support and change to your physical, mental, and emotional well-being. Massage has become an alternative to unexplained pain, discomfort, and tension deep in the body. The bodywork community and other healing disciplines recognize the body's inherent healing potential.

Our healing wisdom comes from deep within and, given the opportunity, has proven time and time again the information that the layers of anatomy hold. This is an excellent time to heal the body, unresolved traumas, and psychological and spiritual blocks that have occurred in our lives.

The body and mind are deeply intertwined. My goal in this book is to deepen your understanding of the mind-body connection in regards to TMJ. There are no known causes for this disorder. Opening your awareness and looking at all the knowledge that is available with this disorder will help you manage your symptoms.

We all have the same anatomy but are unique in how we express our stress, emotions, and psyche. So our level of tension and pain may vary from person to person.

Massage is a technique whose effects are measurable. If allowed, results can enhance your entire being. Pain tells a story, and we will discuss different types of pain and modalities in massage therapy that can work for you at home. My goal with this book is to give you some measurable massage techniques, to help you shift your awareness, and to teach you how to manage your symptoms associated with TMJ.

My clients have asked me over the years to put this routine in an understandable form so they can prevent further symptoms from recurring, work with their children, relieve the tension and pain associated with wearing braces, lessen the tension in the jaw, drain anesthesia after dental visits, and reduce headaches associated with TMJ. My mission statement is helping others to help themselves!

So here it is! We made it happen! Enjoy!

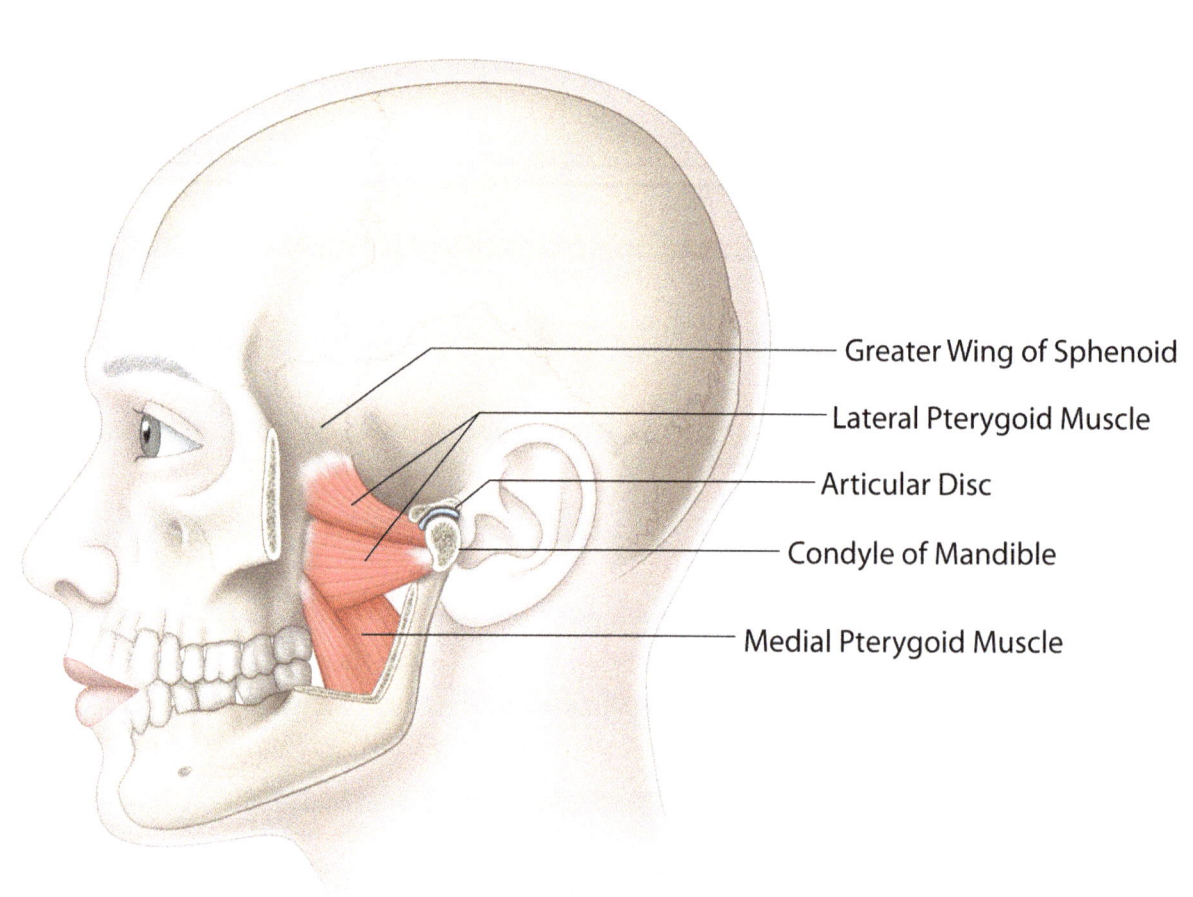

Greater Wing of Sphenoid

Lateral Pterygoid Muscle

Articular Disc

Condyle of Mandible

Medial Pterygoid Muscle

Articular disc

TEMPOROMANDIBULAR JOINT (TMJ) ANATOMY

The temporomandibular joint (TMJ) is made up of the temporal bone, the mandible/jawbone, and the articular disc that is attached to the retrodiscal tissue and sandwiched between two synovial membranes. Synovial membranes are like waterbeds. They line joints and tendon sheaths. Movement occurs in a smooth fluid motion when the membrane is intact.

The temporal bone is where your inner ear is located. Just forward of the ear is the mandibular fossa/indentation that holds the condyles, the rounded ends of the mandible.[1] Ligaments hold the bones together. They are tensile strong and not elastic,[2] so these fibers do not generate pain. The articular disc is attached to the posterior condyle, which carries the disc with it when opening and closing the mouth.[3]

Disc displacement occurs when the disc becomes lodged forward of the condyle and cannot reestablish the connection with the disc. Popping and clicking sounds are associated with disc displacement. Dental splints are usually fitted for this condition. However, muscles play a huge role in misalignment due to tension and trigger points in the muscles.[4]

The articular disc is made up of collagen fibers but is not supplied with blood vessels or a nerve supply. So pain is not generated from the disc. However, the retrodiscal tissue that the disc is attached to becomes compressed between the bones after disc displacement, and inflammation can occur. This tissue is supplied with blood vessels and nerve endings and fed by the synovial membranes. When it becomes damaged, it becomes a major contributor of TMJ pain.[5]

Keeping it simple, let's put it together. When the mouth fully opens, the retrodiscal tissue fully lengthens, and the disc and condyle move forward on the retrodiscal tissue. In a perfect world,

---

[1] David G. Simons, Janet G. Travell, and Lois S. Simons, *Myofascial and Dysfunction Upper Extremities*, vol. 1 (Philadelphia: Williams and Wilkins, 1982), 173.

[2] Steven R. Olmos, DDS, *Functional Anatomy and TM Pathology*, 6.

[3] David G. Simons, Janet G. Travell, and Lois S. Simons, *Myofascial Pain and Dysfunction Upper Extremities*, 173.

[4] Clair Davies and Amber Davies, *The Trigger Point Therapy Workbook*, 3rd ed. (New Harbinger Publications, 2013), 81.

[5] Steven R. Olmos, DDS, *Functional Anatomy and TM Pathology*, 4.

they should slide back again and sit in the mandibular fossa. But if the disc becomes displaced in the forward position, the condyle will return to the joint without the disc and compress the retrodiscal tissue between the two bones. Over time, this irritation to the tissue can create a lot of inflammation and pain.

The next time the mouth opens, the condyle will move forward and try to reconnect to the disc. If this attempt fails, you will hear the popping and clicking when the condyle tries to reposition with the disc. This repetitive striving to reconnect creates trigger points in the muscles, misalignment of the jaw, disc displacement by reducing movement of the condyle, misalignment of the teeth, restricted mouth opening and closing, and grinding, clenching, and lockjaw. [6]

Relief is on the way. Are you ready to change your situation?

---

[6] Clair Davies and Amber Davies, The Trigger Point Therapy Workbook, 3rd ed., 6.

EDUCATE YOURSELF

Knowledge is power. The more you know, the easier it is to get to the root of the problem. I have been grateful time and time again for the knowledge I have gained by becoming a massage therapist. Anatomy is concrete. You can feel it, touch it, and manipulate it.

This quick reference guide will help you to evaluate your pain. You will learn

- the basic anatomy of the TMJ;
- the five muscles of mastication/chewing;
- the trigger points and their referral pain patterns specific to each muscle;
- massage techniques to release tension in the muscles;
- which muscles contribute to clenching, grinding, lockjaw, popping, and clicking; and
- which muscles contribute to disc displacement and misalignment.

Your working knowledge of this routine increases your conversational skills with other practitioners and empowers you in your quest for pain relief. Using this routine between visits with other practitioners enhances the healing process. Let your dentist, orthodontist, massage therapist, cranial sacral therapist, and other health-care providers know you are working with this routine.

Learning how to apply massage techniques correctly will effectively reduce your pain and symptoms associated with TMJ. With repetition, you will develop a sensitivity to your touch. You will learn to adjust your pressure when contacting tissues. Work gently and slowly instead of forcing your way through the tissues to get results. This will help to eliminate pain and alignment issues. Working slowly allows you to evaluate tissues for knots, taut bands, and inflammation/fullness in the area. If you push too hard, you will elicit a guarding response in the tissues. Muscles become tighter, blood flow decreases, and your pain level will go up. So back out. Wait for the tissues to soften and relax. We all have the same anatomy, but how our symptoms arise depends on our past and present physical, emotional, and mental experiences. We are unique in our own way!

UNDERSTANDING PAIN

Pain tells a story. Muscle aches and pain are two of the top complaints of people seeking help from massage therapy. Let's look at this a bit further. Did the pain come on suddenly or gradually over time, reducing your activity level and range of motion? Did a certain event or lifestyle change upset your mental or emotional state, and did you have trouble bouncing back? How do you handle stress?

Pain is described as acute or chronic in massage therapy. Acute pain is sharp and severe and comes on suddenly. Symptoms include heat, redness, swelling, and inflammation. Consult your health care provider, and do not work in these areas if you are experiencing any of these symptoms. The modality commonly used for acute pain in massage therapy is ice. I cannot say enough about ice in the first twenty-four to forty-eight hours after an injury. It helps to reduce inflammation dramatically. After an injury, use ice every hour on the hour for the first eight to twelve hours. The decrease in pain can be dramatic. The acronym RICE (rest, ice, compress, and elevate the injured area) is basic injury first aid.

Chronic pain is pain and inflammation in the soft tissues of the body. This includes muscles, ligaments, tendons, and fascia. Fascia covers every organ, muscle, blood vessel, nerve, and bone in the body. It is avascular, meaning it has low blood supply but is highly nerve innervated. Myofascial pain is one of the major causes of unexplained pain in the body. If an injury is not the cause of pain, the underlying chronic issues that have been weakening an area over time rise to the occasion, eliciting an acute pain response. The body asks for immediate attention. Ice an area if it is sore. If you experience stiffness, alternating ice and heat will reduce any inflammation and increase the blood flow. Alternating this combination can help to increase the healing process in the tissues. Consult your doctor before application.

Educate yourself about fascia. The medical community is starting to acknowledge this amazing tissue and how it affects chronic pain. Some practitioners are specifically trained in myofascial release techniques and would appreciate someone doing this trigger point therapy self-care routine between visits.

Nutrition, hydration, and health of the gut have been helpful in reducing chronic pain symptoms, decreasing stress levels, and improving the health of the immune system in my clients.[7] I have witnessed an improvement after they have incorporated these changes.

An excellent way to lower stress levels and relax the body is through breathing techniques. They are simple, inexpensive, and effective and can be done around any person, place, or thing that upsets you. Breathing techniques help the nervous system to lower the complex stress (inflammation) response in the body. As you practice, the body will begin to entrain to the effects and start breathing for you when you come under stress. It is amazing to experience your body talking to you.

Give it a try! Start inhaling and exhaling through your nose. Focus inward, and follow your breath for a few minutes. If your mind wanders off, bring it back to your breathing and continue. The mind will really try to sabotage you, so keep working with the cycle. Breathe, refocus, and breathe. Build up to five minutes. After five minutes, you should feel more open and relaxed. Keep the breathing going, and see if you can deepen the cycles into the abdomen. Repeat for another five minutes, breathing slowly and evenly.

My clients have done very well with using breathing techniques to manage pain levels. If you experience a lot of negative thoughts, this will help rewire your brain.

With each negative thought, start the breathing, refocusing, and breathing cycle. Deepen the breathing into the abdomen, and affirm that you want to release the pattern in you that causes this negative thought process.

The body knows how to heal itself. So with a few simple techniques, you can start to have a conversation with your body and shift your awareness. The physiological benefits are pretty amazing. Prove to yourself that you can control your stress and reduce your pain.

You can deal with physical trauma in the same way. Use basic first aid for injuries, and include the breathing techniques to integrate the physical forces trapped in the tissues by a trauma.

---

[7] Dr. Gary Kaplan, DO, *Total Recovery: Breaking the Cycle of Chronic Pain and Depression* (New York: Rodale Books, 2014).

You can deal with emotional and mental traumas the same way. Breathing techniques can help the nervous system to relax and integrate the psychological issues so they do not stay trapped in the tissues.

In other words, you will reduce the fight-or-flight response and freeze response in the tissues. Don't be afraid to find a health-care professional to help you with these issues. Overwhelming situations need support from someone who can hold the space for you to heal. Clarity will come with support.

The relief you can feel when you stop carrying around emotional and mental issues can be life-changing. In my craniosacral training, unresolved traumas are major contributors to chronic pain.

MIND-BODY CONNECTION

Massage therapy recognizes the direct mind-body connection. In working with people who have chronic pain over the years, I've found clients show improvement when they are able to connect to unresolved traumas trapped in the tissues. In massage therapy, we call this *emotional mapping*. From birth, we store our experiences in the tissues of the body. The compressions from birth, if not resolved, organize around this chaos and shape our physical, emotional, psychological, and social states structurally in the tissues of the body. The relationships with our parents and caretakers, along with our reactions to our environments, become wired in our nervous systems and can stay with us into adulthood. It sounds grim, but once you think about why you react to certain people or situations and wonder why you just did or said something so off-kilter, you can take a step back and work with this fresh paradigm. Tissue memory can be released. Body-centered therapies are excellent for making this connection.[8]

As babies, we are working from the reptilian brain, which reacts to our world. We need the safety and encouragement of our families to build a strong sense of self and to feel safe in our environment. We look into the eyes of our parents for reassurance and their responses to our needs. If they are angry and/or depressed and don't feed or change us when we need something, our nervous systems respond with fight-or-flight/freeze response. Those are the only resources we have as infants. Since our analytical brain isn't developed, we must process everything from the reptilian brain.

Stop and think about that. How would your life present itself if you were constantly reacting to your environment? Have you ever asked yourself, *What was I thinking?* after a confrontation or conversation? As we get older, our stress levels mimic those early times. So being aware of your reaction to different situations and people can help you to integrate those old stimuli.

The birthing process physically traps a lot of compressed energy and freezes it in layers of tissue. The mandible, for instance, takes on a lot of dragging forces during the birth process. We carry that physical stress for the rest of our lives. As we grow older, we start to develop our speech

---

[8] Michael Kern, *Wisdom in the Body: The Craniosacral Approach to Essential Health* (Berkeley, Calif.: North Atlantic Books, 2001), 237.

and begin to communicate. What happens when our caregivers and parents tell us that we are to be seen and not heard?[9] Well, those looks, statements, and judgments are stored deeply in the nervous system on their way into the subconscious mind.

So how do we recognize those unresolved traumas? This list comes from my years of experience working with birth trauma and TMJ. Emotions drive pain levels.[10] So as you are working with this routine, allow yourself to let go! Quiet your mind, and allow the tissues to talk to you. You might be surprised with what you find.

How do we recognize this complexity?

Guarding ourselves shows a fight-or-flight response in the nervous system, so we grind, clench, overreact with anger and frustration, tense up, or become anxious. Or if there were abuse, we shut down and slither away, frozen in the hopelessness of the experience. Here are a few guidelines to help you recognize unresolved issues trapped in the nervous system.[11]

Sympathetic agitation feels like this:

- You have trouble sleeping or grind your teeth while you are asleep.
- You have restlessness.
- You have muscle tension.
- You grind or clench your teeth.
- You have a rapid heartbeat.
- You have an attraction to dangerous situations.
- You have anger or frustration.
- You are quick to react (short-tempered).
- You have feelings of fearfulness or paranoia.

---

[9] Louise L. Hay, *You Can Heal Your Life* (Carlsbad, Calif.: Hay House, 1999), 201.

[10] Bessel van der Kolk, MD, *The Body Keeps the Score: Brain, Mind, and Body in the Healing of Trauma* (New York: Penguin Group, 2014), 75.

[11] Peter Levine, *Waking the Tiger: Healing Trauma* (Berkeley, Calif.: North Atlantic Books, 1997), 147–149.

Parasympathetic shutdown feels like this:

- You are spacey, unfocused, or forgetful.
- You feel helplessness or hopelessness.
- Your digestion is slow.
- You are depressed.
- You are listless.
- You have chronic fatigue.

Take your time to focus inward. Stop what you are doing and refocus. Give yourself five minutes with breathing to shift the physiological reaction happening in the body. Let it go! Get busy doing something else. This will allow the brain to let go of the old pattern and rewire a new one. Body-centered meditation, yoga, and breathing exercises are a few suggestions to help integrate and manage stress.

You might need the help of a professional to hold space for you. Once you understand and can relax into the process, it's easier to do on your own. I encourage you to seek a safe, supportive health care professional who understands trauma and can help you allow these feelings to emerge, integrate, and heal.

Empower yourself. Live the life you desire.

MASSAGE TECHNIQUES

Trigger point therapy is a massage technique that involves the application of ischemic pressure to tender muscle tissue in order to relieve pain in other parts of the body. It may also be called myofascial (myo, meaning muscle, fascial meaning connective tissue). Both muscles and fascia can have trigger points. The trigger point technique can release both tissues.

Myofascial release is a technique that releases fascia and you will learn simple techniques in this routine.

Fascia has three layers.

Superficial layer is associated with the skin.

Deep layers are associated with muscles, bones, nerves and blood vessels.

Visceral layer which covers the organs and holds them in place.

You will be working with the superficial layers to start. As you repeat the routine, the body will let you into the deeper layers.

This is a non-force technique. Feel for a tight area in the muscle you are working, stretch the skin slightly, and wait patiently for signs of release. (The tissue under the skin will move under your stretch.) Follow the movement of the release in whatever direction it takes you, until the movement stops. Repeat if you feel tension. Trigger point any knots, tender spots, and/or taut bands. Use the trigger point illustrations as your guide.

Once you get a feel for this technique, you can use it all over the body.

Skin rolling is lifting the skin and rolling it between two fingers.

Stripping is sliding fingers in the direction of the muscle fibers to increase fresh circulation to an area. This will give you a chance to locate trigger points, knots, and taut bands.

Signs of release are when the trigger points start to release and the muscles relax. You will feel different sensations that include warming, softening, lengthening, widening, tingling, and feeling of spaciousness. Signs of release for fascia include a softening, gliding movement under your fingers, warming, and tingling. Releases can be felt all over the body, regardless of where you are working.

Ischemic compression is the term used to describe the application of pressure to a trigger point. Use your fingertip or a cotton swab to locate and apply pressure to a hypersensitive area in the muscle. **The illustrations show specific locations in the muscles.**

Muscle	Function	Cause and Effect of Active Trigger Points
Masseter	Closing the jaw Biting Chewing	Grinding Clenching Restricting opening Sinusitis Tooth hypersensitivity (too hot or cold) Stuffiness in ear Itching in the ear Head-forward posture Whiplash Dental work Tinnitus[12]

Temporalis	Closing the jaw Retrusion of mandible Chewing	Restricting the opening of the mouth Tooth sensitivity Malocclusion Clenching Grinding Gum chewing Thumb sucking after infancy Dental work[13]
Digastric	Opening jaw Retrusion of mandible	Mouth breathing Grinding Clenching Difficulty swallowing Tenderness in throat, tongue, and palate[14]
Medial Pterygoid	Closing the jaw Assisting in chewing	Restricting the opening of the mouth Preventing the Eustachian tube from opening Grinding Clenching Sucking thumb after infancy Chewing gum Emotional stress Prolonged opening of the mouth during dental work Pain biting down Pain in throat Swallowing[15]

Lateral Pterygoid	Opening the jaw Pulling mandible out of the joint, moving the jaw from side to side	Number-one source of pain in TMJ Locking of the jaw Disc displacement Malocclusion Popping Clicking Mouth breathing Sinusitis Prolonged dental work Pain biting down[16]

[12] Clair Davies and Amber Davies, *The Trigger Point Therapy Workbook*, 3rd ed., 82–86.

[13] David G. Simons, Janet G. Travell, and Lois S. Simons, *Myofascial Pain and Dysfunction*, vol. 1 (Philadelphia: Williams and Wilkins, 1982), 223,231, 236, 252, 260, 264.

[14] David G. Simons, Janet G. Travell, and Lois S. Simons, *Myofascial Pain and Dysfunction*, vol. 1 (Philadelphia: Williams and Wilkins, 1982), 223,231, 236, 252, 260, 264.

[15] Ibid.

[16] Clair Davies and Amber Davies, *The Trigger Point Therapy Workbook*, 3rd ed.

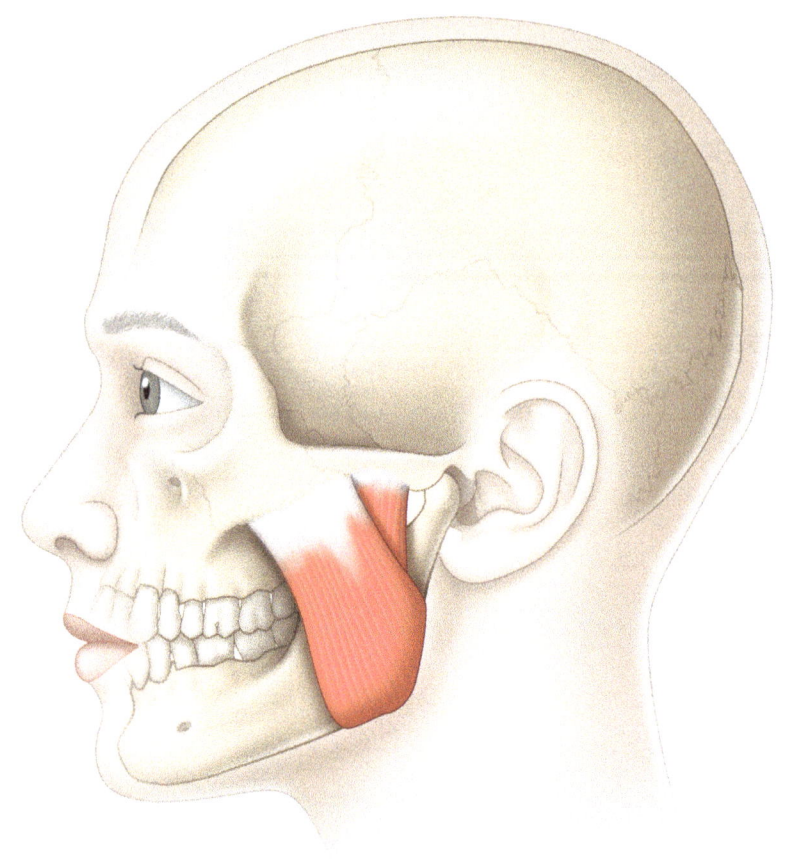

Masseter Muscle

Action: closes the jaw, assists in chewing and biting down.

Dysfunction: grinding, clenching, sinusitis, tooth sensitivity, itching, stuffiness, tinnitus in the ear.

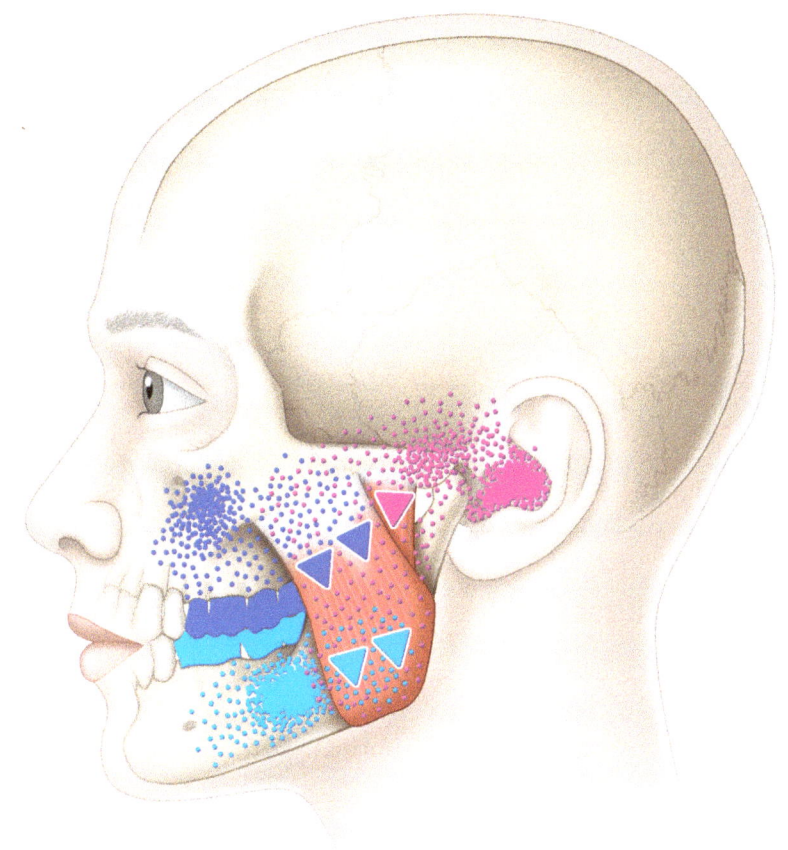

Masseter Trigger Points

- Strip muscle
- Trigger point

NOTES

MASSAGE TECHNIQUES FOR MASSETER

Warm up muscles using skin rolling and stripping before doing trigger points.

Masseter—Large

- Skin rolling: Use one finger on the inside of the cheek and the other on the outside. Pinch and roll between fingers. Work from top to bottom and side to side.
- Stripping. This technique is a gliding motion using your thumb, knuckle, or fingertips. Follow the direction of the muscle fibers. Start at the mandible, and work toward the cheekbone. The illustrations show the fibers of the muscles nicely.
- Find the trigger points in the illustration, and the most tender spot is where you will start.
- Hold trigger points for one to five minutes. When I work a trigger point, I wait for the pulsing to start and stop. This resets the muscle length, and the results are more complete. Signs of release will feel spacious, like there is more room in your mouth, warmth, tingling.
- Work on the next trigger point. Repeat until all trigger points are released. If tender, only work as many trigger points as comfortable. Results will come in time.
- Stripping after trigger points will help remove toxins. Relax!

Masseter—Small

The small masseter is directly in front of the ear.

- Skin rolling: The small masseter can feel as hard as a bone and be very tender. So you might want to find the trigger point first and then do the massage techniques. Use your common sense here! Try both ways of releasing the muscle, and see what your body likes best.
- Stripping: at an angle. Illustration shows fiber direction. Cross fiber friction. Work against the grain over the ropey edge of the muscle.
- Trigger point: for one to five minutes or until pulsing starts and stops. Wait for signs of release.

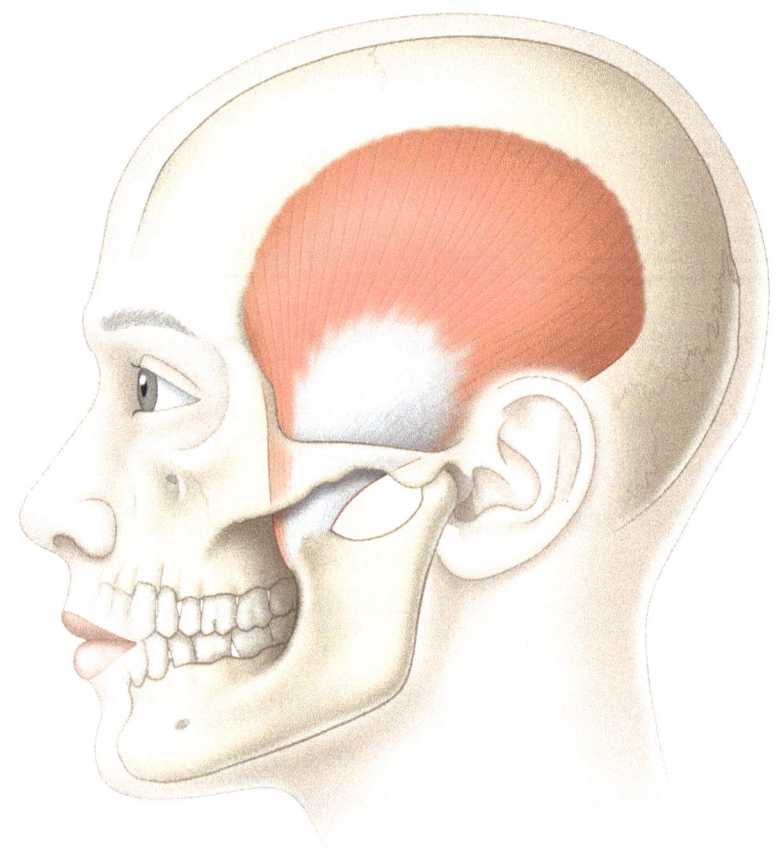

Temporalis Muscle

Action: closes the jaw, assists in chewing and in biting, and retrusion (backward) movement of mandible.

Dysfunction: tooth sensitivity, clenching, grinding, malocclusion, and restricting of the mouth opening.

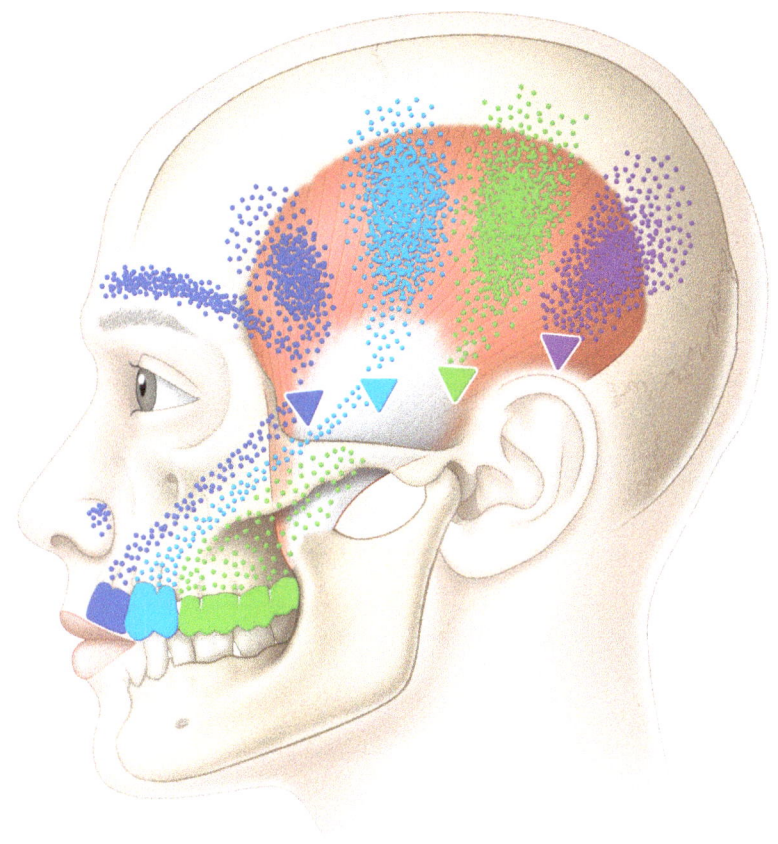

Temporalis Trigger Points

- Myofascial release
- Strip muscle
- Trigger point

NOTES

MASSAGE TECHNIQUES FOR TEMPORALIS MUSCLE

Locate the temporalis tendon. Slowly start opening and closing the jaw with small movements, fingers above your cheekbone, just over the tmj. You will feel it moving under your fingers when you open and close the jaw. Once you have found the tendon, use your fingertips to traction the skin and tendon upward and hold. Wait for signs of release.

Option: This move is great if you place your elbows on the table and let the weight of your head hang from your fingertips while holding the upward traction on the tendon. Repeat for the muscle (next technique).

Traction the muscle: spreading all your fingers wide across the entire muscle, above the ear. Traction the muscle upwards, and hold for signs of release.

Traction the scalp: place fingers as close to your scalp and gently traction the roots of your hair outwards. Loosens fascia on the cranium (myofascial technique). Wait for signs of release.

Stripping: temporalis has three different fiber directions. (See illustration.) Strip in the fiber direction. Feel for taut band, knots, or tender spots.

Trigger Point

Trigger point muscle. Hold for one to five minutes or until pulsing starts and stops. Wait for signs of release.

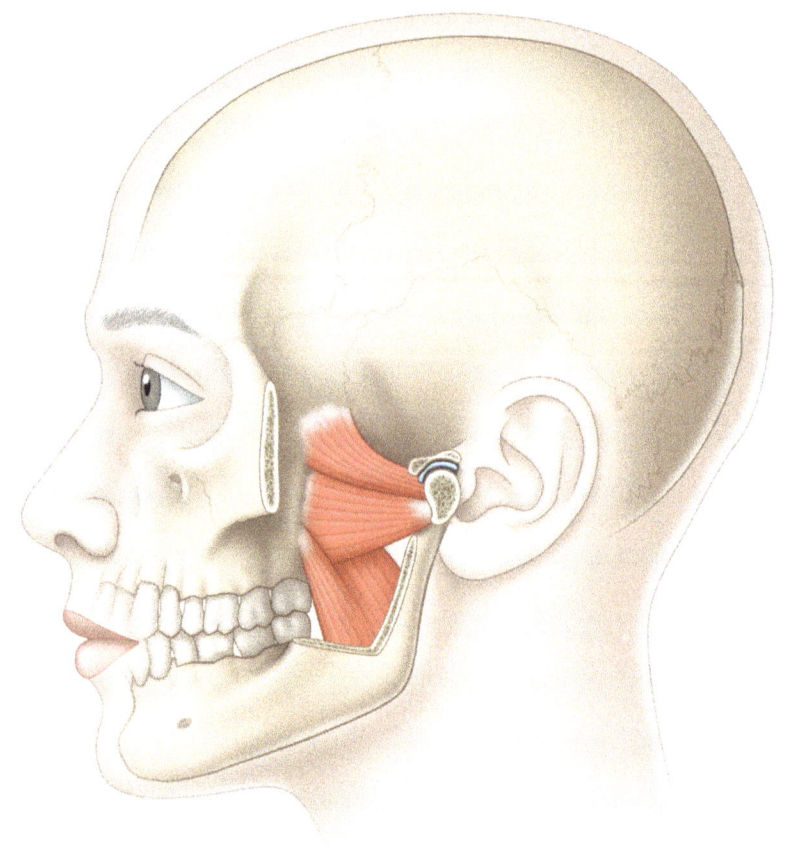

Medial Pterygoid Muscle

Action: aids in chewing and helps to close the jaw

Dysfunction: grinding, clenching, restricting of the opening of the mouth after dental visits, and pain in throat

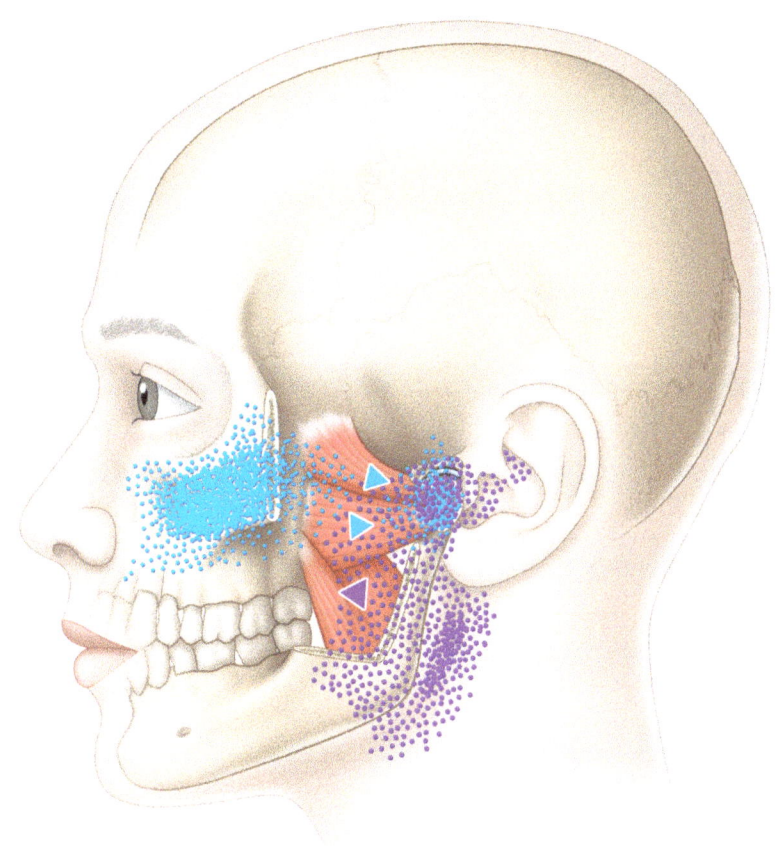

Medial Pterygoid Trigger Points

- Trigger point
- Strip muscle behind molars to corner of jaw.

NOTES

MASSAGE TECHNIQUES FOR MEDIAL PTERYGOID

Guide your finger along the bottom of your upper teeth, past your last molar, until you feel a vertical band. The muscle runs behind the upper teeth to the inside corner of the mandible.

With jaw and tongue relaxed, strip the vertical band from the upper teeth down to the bottom teeth with a "C" motion. This muscle feels hard like a bone if tight. Trigger point. Repeat three times if not too tender.

Lying down can help with the gag reflex and drooling.

External attachment is under the corner of jaw. Muscle will feel like a knot.

Caution! The carotid artery is behind the corner of the mandible. You will feel a pulse in this area. Do not press on the pulse. Work around it, not on it.

Skin rolling: gently work the side of your finger under the mandible. Start at the chin, and work back to the corner of the mandible and around corner of the jaw up to the ear. Gently roll your finger into and away from the jaw bone. This is a small move. Work around the corner and up the back of the mandible gently. Always check for the pulse of the carotid artery.

Trigger point: Hook your thumb or finger up under the corner of the mandible and gently work the muscle next to the bone until you find the trigger point. Hold the point, wait for signs of release, and relax!

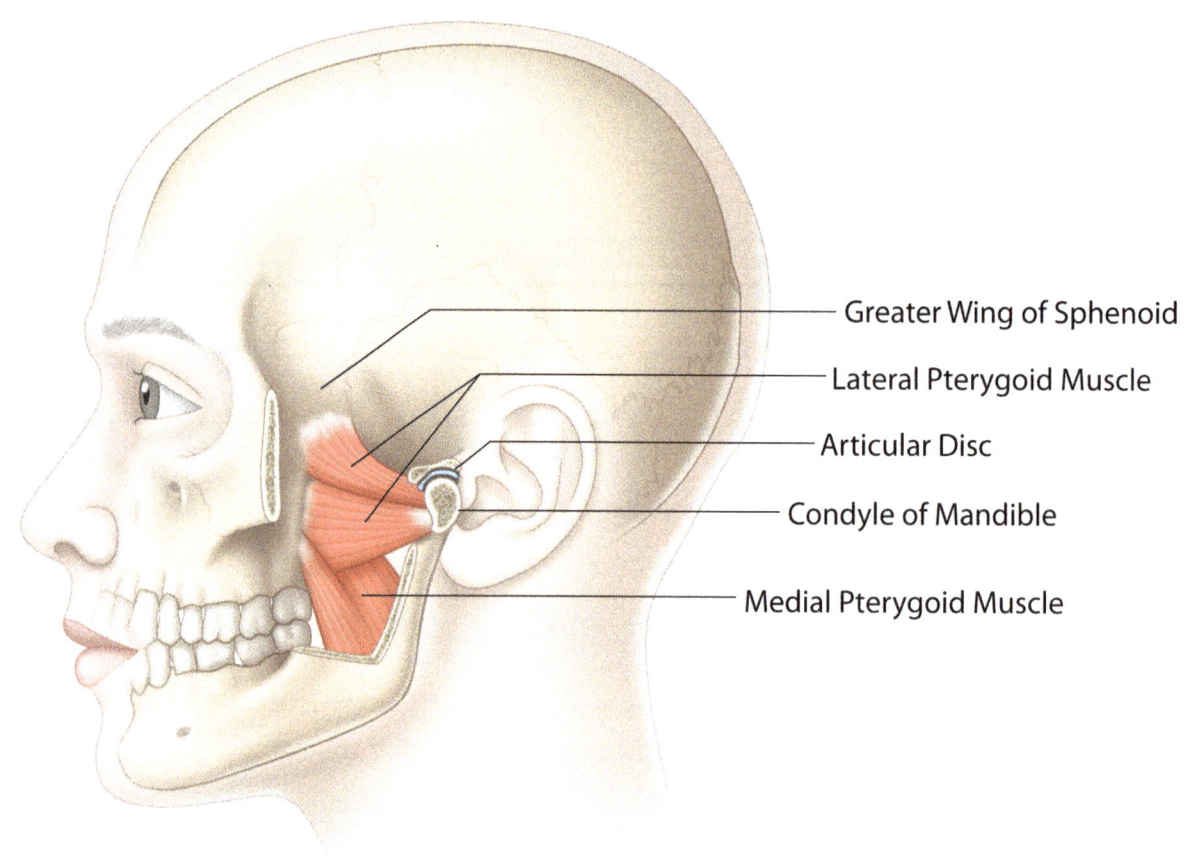

Greater Wing of Sphenoid

Lateral Pterygoid Muscle

Articular Disc

Condyle of Mandible

Medial Pterygoid Muscle

Lateral Pterygoid

Action: opening the mouth, moving the mandible forward and out of the joint, and moving the jaw from side to side.

Dysfunction: number-one source of pain in TMJ, lockjaw, popping and clicking sounds, sinusitis, tension after dental visits, malocclusion, trouble breathing through the nose/mouth breathing.

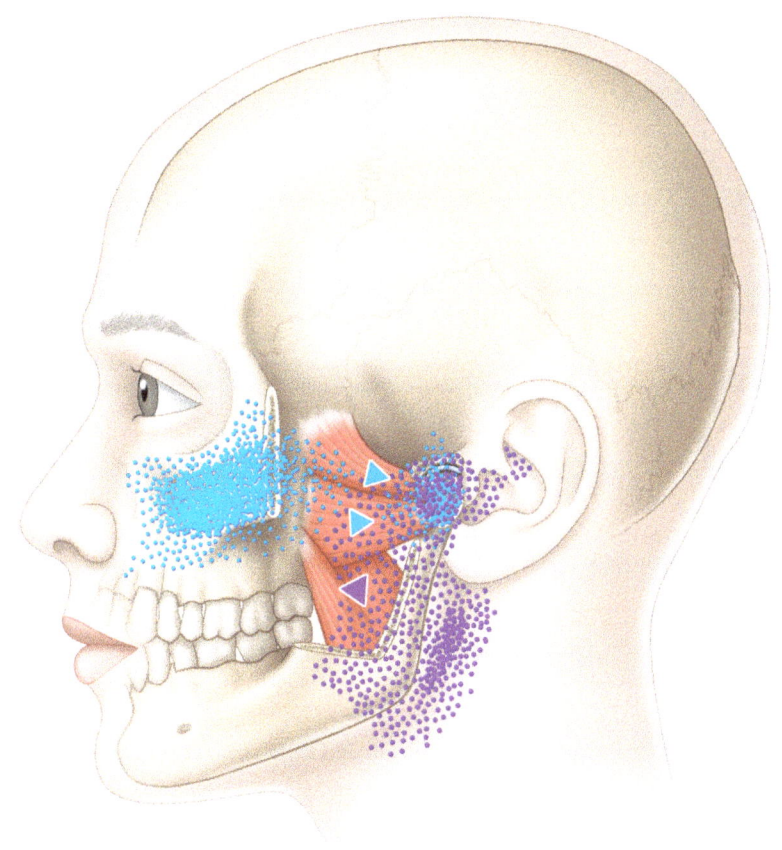

Lateral Pterygoid Trigger Points

- • Trigger point
- • Stripping muscle

NOTES

MASSAGE TECHNIQUES FOR LATERAL PTERYGOID

I encourage you to find patience with these next two muscles. They can be extremely painful when you first start this routine.

When you first start trying to locate lateral pterygoid, you will wonder if you are in the right place, that is, if what you palpate is actually the muscle or a bone. Remember, you are not used to visually seeing this muscle, like you can in your arm or leg. There is no proprioception of this muscle to your knowledge. By now, you have learned some anatomy and worked with other muscles so you are one step closer to finding it.

Trigger point the muscle before the stripping technique.

Inferior Head

Guide your finger or pinky finger along the gum line of your upper teeth until you reach the last tooth/molar. Keep going until you sink into a soft fleshy hollow. Direct your finger upwards, and slowly open and close your jaw. You will feel the inferior head of the lateral pterygoid moving on the condyle of the mandible. This muscle is short and strong. Relax your tongue and jaw! This is very important to help reduce pain and relax the muscle. Find trigger point. Repeat. Wait for pulsing to start and stop and you feel signs of release.

Lying down can help with the gag reflex and drooling.

Bite down on your finger to feel the trigger point. Use a cotton swab if the mouth opening is small. Locate the trigger point, hold until pulsing starts and stops, and repeat if you can tolerate. Wait for signs of release and relax!

Strip: the muscle after trigger point technique(optional). This muscle is very sore on most people, so very light pressure is all you need. Icing can help afterward. Rest and ice for a few days if really sore, before and after. An ice cube in a sandwich baggy works well. As you release the trigger points completely, pain will subside, and movement in the jaw will increase.

Superior Head

Locating lateral pterygoid: on the outside of your mouth, place your fingers over the TMJ. Open and close the mouth to locate the joint. (See the illustration). Now find the hollow between the condyles of the mandible(open jaw). You will be able to feel the muscle moving. Use a fingertip in this hollow will strip and trigger point the lateral superior head. Trigger point both sides of the mouth to keep your bite even.

Trigger point: Inside the mouth(between teeth and jaw). Open and close to find the superior head, just above where you were working with the medial pterygoid. Roll your fingertip left and right to strip.

Optional: Use a cotton swab, if necessary. If sore, lighten pressure but don't move off the point. Hold the trigger point until pulsing starts and stops. Wait for signs of release. Ice and rest a day or two between routines.

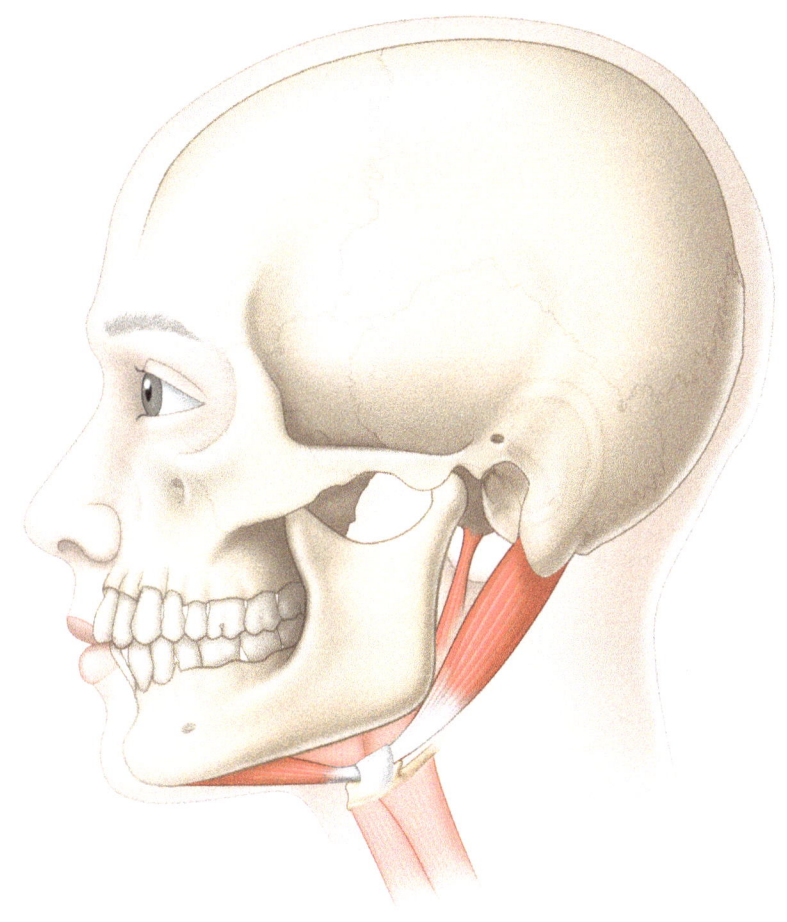

Digastric Muscle

Action: aids in swallowing, opening the jaw, and retrusion of the jaw (backward).

Dysfunction: grinding, clenching, mouth breathing, and tenderness in the throat.

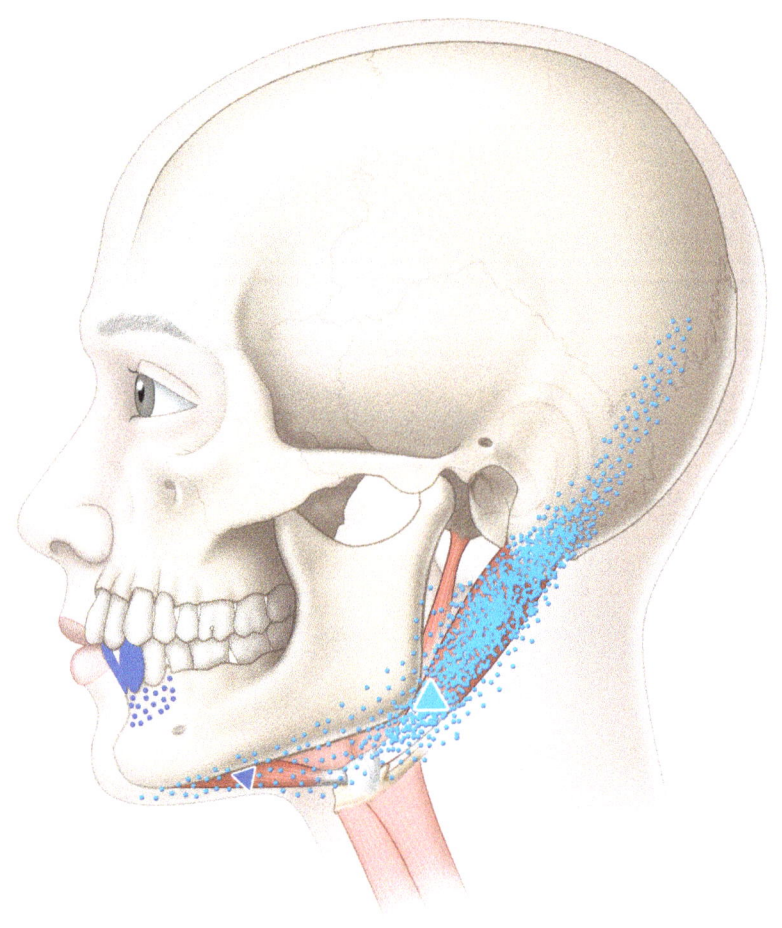

Digastric Trigger Points

- Trigger point
- Strip muscle from chin to angle of jaw.

NOTES

MASSAGE TECHNIQUES FOR DIGASTRIC MUSCLES

The action of the muscle is secondary to other muscles, but it's worth adding to the routine. Digastric and stylohyoid help to stabilize and line up the hyoid bone. The posterior belly attaches to the bump (mastoid process) behind your ear. The anterior attachment is on the inside of the chin. In the illustration, the digastric is the wider muscle. The thinner muscle is the stylohyoid muscle. These muscles help make up the floor of the mouth.

CAUTION! Gently press in this hollow. A slight widening is all you are trying to accomplish. Deep pressure can irritate a nerve.

Massage under the chin and trigger point, the anterior bellies.

Using stripping, feel for the groove between the mastoid process and the ear. It is a very small space, just perfect for your fingertip. Gently move your jaw forward and backward with small movements to find the muscle. Once you have found it, start slowly and lightly to rotate your fingertip in that groove. If it is tender, lighten your pressure. Wait for signs of release.

Caution! There is a boney attachment(point) that the stylohyoid attaches to. Light pressure is all that is needed here. If tender, use light pressure, a little work will go a long way. You won't trigger point the posterior belly.

Use stripping under the chin. The anterior bellies have a trigger point. Start by stroking your fingers from the chin to the Adam's apple. See if you can feel the hyoid bone between these two points. If not, that is okay. The two muscle bellies will feel ropey.

Trigger point the anterior muscle bellies under the chin. Wait for signs of release. Relax!

GLOSSARY

Anterior: This is located toward the front of the body.

Articular disc: This connective tissue disc acts as a cushion between the two bones. It's collagen tissue with no blood or nerve supply. It does not produce pain.

Attachment: the point where muscles or tendons attach to a bone.

Bilateral: This means two muscles, one on each side of the body.

Digastric: This is a suprahyoid muscle that makes up the floor of the mouth and assists in opening the jaw and swallowing.

Disc displacement: This is forward dislocation of the articular disc. The disc locks forward on the retrodiscal tissue and doesn't return to its original position between the two bones. The jaw locks and clicks when opening.

External: These are muscles on the outside of the head.

Fascia: These bands of tissue under the skin interconnect all tissues, muscles, bones, organs, and nerves.

Internal: These muscles are on the inside of the mouth.

Ischemic compression: pressure applied to a tender spot in a muscle, forcing the blood out of the area. When released a new surge of fresh oxygenated blood floods into an area. Relieves referral pain and local pain in muscles and fascia.

Lateral pterygoid: This muscle assists in closing the jaw, pulling the disc forward, and facilitating the rotary motion of chewing.

Malocclusion: This is misalignment of the teeth, that is, teeth not fitting together correctly.

Mandible: This is the jawbone.

Masseter: This muscle closes the mouth and assists in biting and clamping down with the teeth.

Mastication: This means chewing.

Maxilla: These two bones in the mouth hold the upper teeth and maxillary sinuses. They meet with the palate and sphenoid bone and are used as a guide for the internal muscles.

Massage techniques: These are techniques applied with your hands or fingers to release muscles and fascia in the body. Included in this book will be skin rolling, stripping, and trigger points.

Medial pterygoid: This internal muscle assists in chewing motion and closing and protruding of the jaw (e.g., an underbite).

Myofascial release: myo(meaning muscle) and fascial meaning connective tissue. Technique releases fascia and trigger points.

Posterior: This means toward the back of the body.

Protrusion: This is forward movement of the mandible (e.g., underbite).

Referral pain: pain that is felt in another area of the body away from the trigger point(cause).

Retrodiscal tissue: This connective tissue attaches the disc to the temporal fossa, allowing the disc to stretch forward when the mouth opens. It holds the disc in place as it moves over the condyle. This tissue is supplied by blood and nerves; therefore, it is a major source of pain in the joint.

Retrusion: This is backward movement of the mandible.

Skin rolling: This myofascial release technique involves lifting the skin and rolling it between two fingers.

Stripping: This is a massage technique where you start sliding your fingers from one end of the muscle to the other in the direction of the muscle fibers. (See illustrations for fiber direction.)

Temporalis: This is a muscle on the side of the head where the action is to close the jaw.

Temporomandibular joint (TMJ): This joint is made up of two bones and a disc (temporal bone, articular disc, and condyle of the mandible). It is responsible for movement of the joint.

Trauma: This is a physical injury or emotional, psychological event that elicits an overwhelming response of shock that cannot be discharged from the nervous system. The unresolved issues become trapped in the tissues, bone, and psyche.

Trigger point: This is hypersensitivity in the muscle or fascial tissue. Trigger points can include knots, taut bands, and tender spots that refer pain to other areas of the body.

RESOURCES

Chi Nei Tsang Institute. *Visceral Manipulation*. Berkeley, Calif.

Coomes, Annie, LMT. "Oh My Aching Back." www.cranialsacral.blogspot.com.

Daniluk, Julie, RHN. *Meals That Heal Inflammation: Embrace Healthy Living and Eliminate Pain, One Meal at a Time*. Carlsbad, Calif.: Hay House, 2011.

Clair Davies and Amber Davies, *The Trigger Point Therapy Workbook*, 3rd ed.

Dispensa, Joe. http://www.learn.hayhouseu.com/joedispenza

Durana-Scurlock, Suzanne. *Full Body Presence: Learning to Listen to Your Body's Wisdom*. Novato, Calif.: New World Library, 2011.

Gach, Reed Michael. *Acupressure's Potent Points: A Guide to Self-Care for Common Ailments*. New York: Bantam Books, 1990.

Hay, Louise L. *Heal Your Body*. Carlsbad, Calif.: Hay House 1982, 1984.

Herman, Judith, MD. *Trauma and Recovery*. New York: Basic Books, 1992, 1997.

Kaplan, Gary Dr., DO. *Total Recovery: Breaking the Cycle of Chronic Pain and Depression*. New York: Rodale Books, 2014.

Levine, Peter. *Waking the Tiger: Healing Trauma*. Berkeley, Calif.: North Atlantic Books, 1997.

Chia, Mantak, and Juan Li. *The Inner Structure of Tai Chi: Mastering the Classic Forms of Tai Chi Chi Kung*. Rochester, Vt.: Destiny Books, 2005.

Pert, Candace B. *Molecules of Emotion: Why You Feel The Way You Feel*. New York: Scribner, 1997.

Michael Kern, *Wisdom in the Body: The Craniosacral Approach to Essential Health* (Berkeley, Calif.: North Atlantic Books, 2001), 237.

Louise L. Hay, *You Can Heal Your Life* (Carlsbad, Calif.: Hay House, 1999), 201.

Bessel van der Kolk, MD, *The Body Keeps the Score: Brain, Mind, and Body in the Healing of Trauma* (New York: Penguin Group, 2014), 75.

Olmos Steven DDS, *Functional Anatomy and TMJ Pathology4*
www.dentalacademyofce.com/courses/1445/pdf/functionalanatomy.pdf

ABOUT THE AUTHOR

Annie Coomes is a 1992 graduate of Ball State University with a bachelor's degree in exercise science. She graduated from Colorado Institute of Massage Therapy (CIMT) in Colorado Springs and was certified in craniosacral therapy in Boulder in 2000.

She lives and practices craniosacral therapy in Colorado.

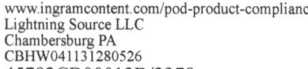